THE IBD ANTI-INFLAMMATORY HEALING DIET

Natural Remedies, Diet Management, and Alkaline Recipes

Rose Annear

Copyright © 2024 Rose Annear

All rights reserved.

ISBN: 9798339011842

CONTENTS

Introduction 7
What Is Inflammatory Bowel Disease (IBD)? 10
Does Diet Have An Impact On IBD? 14
Following an Anti-inflammatory Diet for IBD 18
Handling Flare-ups and Remissions 22
Important Lifestyle Interventions for IBD 26
What to Consider When Choosing Foods 30
Sample Plant-Based Recipes for IBD 33
Conclusion 61

Introduction

Inflammatory bowel disease (IBD for short) is a broad term used to describe the inflammation of the gastrointestinal tract. It specifically refers to conditions like Crohn's disease and ulcerative colitis.

Even though IBD is a chronic and lifelong illness, it is treatable! However, it would be wrong to assume that just eating certain foods can cure the condition; it requires a lot more which encompasses both nutrition and lifestyle interventions.

Having said that, diet plays an important role in the underlying inflammatory processes that lead up to IBD symptoms. Eating the right food can help to manage the disease during flare-ups and periods of remission. More importantly, it can promote recovery.

Due to how unpredictable IBD symptoms can be, this can present a daily challenge for those affected. This is why it's important to understand the intricate relationship between your food choices and gut health, whether you're dealing with ulcerative colitis or Crohn's disease.

While certain foods may worsen our symptoms, others can actually help to calm them and aid healing. The purpose of this book is to help demystify the IBD diet and offer practical tips on various lifestyle changes to ensure you live a more comfortable, active life even while on the road to recovery.

What Is Inflammatory Bowel Disease (IBD)?

As earlier indicated, IBD, which usually includes conditions such as ulcerative colitis and Crohn's disease, is associated with inflammation in the digestive system. Specifically, it affects the lining of the digestive tract.

Ulcerative colitis typically affects the colon and rectum. Crohn's disease, on the other hand, can affect any part of your digestive tract, from your mouth to your anus, and can cause fatigue, diarrhea, abdominal pain, and weight loss.

The Gut and How Digestion Takes Place

The gut is a long tube that runs from the mouth all the way to the anus (i.e., where poop comes out), and includes vital organs such as the esophagus, stomach, and intestines.

The main function of the guy is to break down food, so the body can get the nutrients and energy it requires. In other words, it aids in digestion and absorption of nutrients as well as the excretion of waste products of digestion.

What Digestion Looks Like

Before we get into how IBD affects food and digestion, it will help to get a basic overview of what actually goes on when you eat.

When you put food into your mouth, it goes down through the oesophagus into the stomach. The stomach produces acids that kill germs and churns the food into something like porridge.

Next, the food is passed on through the bowels where it is broken down and nutrients and energy are absorbed from it. Whatever that is left (i.e., anything not absorbed) is pushed further into the large bowel where the liquid is absorbed leaving the remaining solid waste, which is then passed out as poo. Before it's passed out, the poo is stored somewhere in the large bowel known as the rectum.

This whole process can take anywhere from 1 to 4 days or even more depending on the individual or what you ate.

How IBD Affects Food & Digestion

As earlier indicated, IBD interferes with the ability of the body to properly digest food, absorb nutrients, and get rid of waste products. Foods and drinks basically pass through the gastrointestinal tract or digestive system. Ulcerative colitis and Crohn's disease cause the gut to become inflamed.

With Crohn's, the inflammation can occur anywhere in the digestive system, from the mouth to the anus. For instance, if the small bowel is affected, it might prevent proper absorption of nutrients from the food. This results in lower energy levels and lack of essential vitamins and minerals.

With colitis, the inflammation usually occurs in the colon or large bowel. Since it's the job of the colon to absorb water from digested food, when it becomes inflamed, it is no longer able to perform that function properly. This causes you to pass out watery stool, which usually leads to diarrhea.

So, what causes IBD?

IBD can be caused by a number of factors, which may include environmental factors, changes in gut bacteria, genetics, and the reactions that occur in the immune system.

If you have anyone in your family who has (or had) IBD, chances are that you may end up getting it too.

Environmental factors mainly border on your lifestyle, what you eat, and your living conditions. Certain conditions may contribute to the development of the disease, especially in someone who is already at risk.

Does Diet Have An Impact On IBD?

It is not clear whether what you eat can cause IBD but we do know that food can have a direct impact on the gut lining.

Specifically, your diet can affect the balance between harmful and helpful bacteria in your gut. As a result, a poor diet can increase your risk of getting IBD, which includes colitis or Crohn's disease.

This is why what you eat when you have this condition is even more important and the reason is not far-fetched.

A lot of IBD patients often suffer from malnutrition and this can be linked to the reasons already stated, which include poor digestion of food, malabsorption of nutrients from the food, reduced desire to eat, and unintended weight loss. Consequently, this increases the caloric needs of the body, especially when the person is experiencing a flare-up.

The Role of a Nutrient-dense IBD Diet

Since IBD is fueled by inflammation, it only makes sense to follow an anti-inflammatory diet when you're dealing with the condition. This is also known as an IBD-AID diet.

An anti-inflammatory diet can help you manage the symptoms of IBD while aiding recovery. It can also influence the severity and frequency of flare-ups. Specifically, it can induce longer periods of remission.

Having said that, it's important to point out that there's no general one-size-fits-all diet for inflammatory bowel disease. You will need to monitor how each food affects your condition, so you can work out a plan that will minimize your symptoms and promote your gut health.

Having said that, there are certain foods you must avoid or completely cut out from your diet. Some of these include:

- Dairy
- Alcohol
- Fried foods

- Refined sugar
- High-fat foods
- Spicy foods
- Caffeine
- Alcohol
- Prunes
- Raw vegetables and other foods high in insoluble fiber (doesn't dissolve in water) such as cabbage, asparagus, cauliflower, kale, and the skin of an apple
- Foods high in lactose such as cream, cow milk, custard, and ice cream
- Artificial sweeteners and other sweetened beverages
- Energy drinks and sodas
- Creamy sauces
- Oranges and orange juice
- Sugary foods such as cookies, honey, and pastries
- Corn and snack foods made with corn such as nacho chips
- Whole nuts and seeds such as pumpkin seeds and sunflower seeds
- High animal proteins such as red meat and processed meat

In addition to the list above, it's also important to identify other food sensitivities, which may not necessarily cause harm to your body but can potentially trigger a flare-up or worsen IBD symptoms. So, I highly recommend keeping a journal to record personal triggers.

Following an Anti-inflammatory Diet for IBD

As earlier indicated, when dealing with IBD, it usually makes sense to follow an anti-inflammatory diet to help counter the ongoing inflammation in your gut. Having said that, individual plans may differ as trigger foods are not exactly the same for everyone.

An anti-inflammatory diet for IBD is mostly plant-based and especially consists of foods rich in Omega-3, high-quality proteins, and certain fruits and veggies (tolerance may vary). These foods are known to decrease inflammation.

I have included a list of some examples.

What to eat for IBD

Fruits

Cantaloupe

Raspberries

Ripe banana

Honeydew

Applesauce

Blended fruit

Papaya

Watermelon

Avocados

Etc.

Vegetables

Cooked kale

Cooked zucchini

Cooked green beans

Cooked squashes

Cooked carrots

Etc.

Grains

Rice

Oats

Quinoa

Cooked potatoes

Etc.

Nuts and seeds

Almonds

Pine nuts

Pistachios

Walnut

Flaxseed

Sunflower seeds

Etc.

Omega-3 fatty acids rich foods

Mackerel (excluded if you're fully going plant-based)

Salmon (not plant-based)

Tuna (not plant-based)

Walnut butter

Flaxseed oil

Canola oil

Olive oil

NOTE: Besides fruits, most other food options should be cooked and cut into small pieces or blended, especially vegetables, to aid their digestion and absorption in the body. In general, when you have IBD, you should opt for bland, soft foods.

Handling Flare-ups and Remissions

When you have IBD, sometimes, the foods your body tolerates while in remission can become a problem during a flare-up.

One way to minimize this is to identify such foods and avoid them, at least until the symptoms have subsided.

Below are some more additional tips to help you manage a flare-up.

Reduce the size of your meals

Instead of two or three large meals in a day, you may want to break them up into smaller, more frequent meals. This will help your digestive system not to become overburdened.

Avoid trigger foods

I've already said this before. If you notice any food exacerbates your symptoms whenever you eat it during a flare-up, it's best to cut it off from your diet. You may try it again when in remission.

Consume more soluble fiber

During a flare-up, you want to limit your intake of insoluble fibers and focus on low-fiber foods instead.

This is because low-fiber foods are much easier to digest and won't cause a lot of irritation in the guts, especially when you have symptoms like diarrhea and abdominal pain.

In fact, focusing on low-fiber foods alone can help relieve your flare-ups. Foods in this category should be soft and bland. Some examples include:

- Bananas
- Oatmeal
- Applesauce

- Plain cereals
- Mashed potatoes
- Diluted fruit juice
- Canned fruits
- Eggs (non-vegan)
- Fish (non-vegan)

Other examples are fruits without hard exteriors and cooked vegetables.

NB: If you're going to eat fruits, make sure to peel and remove the seeds.

Consume more fluids

Another thing you can do when you have flare-ups is to increase your fluid intake.

This is really important, especially if you're having constipation, incomplete evacuation, or frequent loose stools. It doesn't have to be just water; you can also take smoothies and broth.

Avoid sugary drinks and beverages as well as caffeine.

Aim to drink up to 8 cups of water daily. You can have a smoothie or your own natural fruit juice between meals.

Important Lifestyle Interventions for IBD

In addition to nutrition, it's also important to your lifestyle when dealing with IBD. There are certain lifestyle changes you can make that can help ease your symptoms and lower the chances of a flare-up.

Quit smoking and alcohol

If you don't smoke, this doesn't apply to you, but if you do smoke, then it's probably time to stop.

Smoking makes you vulnerable to many diseases, including IBD, which is why it's often listed as a risk factor. Specifically, for IBD, especially Crohn's disease, it can make your condition more severe and harder to treat.

So, don't let all your dietary efforts go to waste by indulging in cigarettes and other tobacco products or drinking alcohol.

Exercise regularly

In addition to following the Dr Sebi diet, another area you should focus on is getting regular exercise.

Staying active comes with a lot of benefits including building bone and muscle mass, promoting circulation, increasing energy, and strengthening the immune system.

Specifically, for people with IBD, exercise helps to support the proper functioning of the digestive system while improving symptoms such as depression and anxiety.

In terms of exercise to do, it's entirely up to you. It can be something as simple as walking or something more involved such as rowing.

In general, anything low to moderate impact will work just fine as long as it's something you enjoy doing.

The main thing is to stay consistent; ideally, you want to get up to 30 minutes of workout daily for 4-5 days per week.

Reduce stress

As with all other diseases, stress can worsen the symptoms of IBD and even trigger flare-ups.

Besides diet and exercise, one of the ways to help manage stress is through relaxation. I'm talking about things like meditation, yoga and even breathing exercises.

I have listed other options:

- Being in nature
- Journaling
- Getting a massage
- Spending time alone
- Talking to a therapist
- Listening to a favorite song
- Getting organized
- Spending time with friends/family
- Etc.

Get enough sleep

We all need sleep to stay alive and remain efficient, but it's even more important for people with IBD. You should try to get at least 8 hours of sleep every night. If you're having trouble sleeping, then you may need to put more effort into creating the right environment. There are many resources online that can help in this regard.

What to Consider When Choosing Foods

So, how exactly do you know whether a fruit or vegetable is easily digestible or not? Well, you can do that by focusing on three things - the type of food, the texture of the food, and how much you're consuming at a time.

Let's take a closer look at each of these:

Type of food

One of the first things you should always look out for when choosing your food is the type. As I said earlier, there are two types of fiber - soluble and insoluble fiber.

Initially, when treating IBD, you need soluble fiber. So, when choosing your fruits or vegetables, you have to make sure they meet this criterion.

One way to know if the fruit or vegetable is a soluble fiber or not is to drop it into water.

For instance, when you drop some fresh raspberries into a glass of water, they quickly start to disintegrate or dissolve; this means it's a soluble fiber.

In contrast, if a fruit or vegetable doesn't readily dissolve in water, such as the skin of an apple, then it's insoluble fiber. You want to avoid insoluble fiber at first as they can cause more frequent trips to the restroom.

Texture of the food

Another thing you should look at is the texture of the food. Most of the time, it may be better to adjust the texture of the food.

For instance, even though raw kale and blended kale have equal amounts of insoluble fiber, they do not have the same texture.

Specifically, it would be much easier for the body to tolerate blended kale due to its "softness" and tendency to act like soluble fiber as it goes down the intestines.

Likewise, instead of eating raw nuts, opt for nut butters as these are easier to digest.

Amount of food

Finally, don't try to eat too much at once, and if you're already used to large portions, try to reduce it.

Also, avoid eating too many fruits and vegetables at once in one meal as these can increase your trips to the bathroom. Take things slowly and add a little at a time as your body tolerates them.

-

Sample Plant-Based Recipes for IBD

CHAI CHAI DRINK

Ingredients

- One banana
- One cup water
- Half a cup coconut milk
- ¼ tsp ground cinnamon
- ¼ tsp ground ginger
- A pinch of ground cardamom
- One or two medjool dates, pitted
- One tablespoon chia seeds (can be substituted with hemp hearts or ground flax)
- One cup alfalfa sprouts, optional

Instructions

1. Put everything in a blender and puree until smooth. You can add more milk or water depending on whether you want it thicker or thinner.

STRAWBERRY SMOOTHIE

Ingredients

- Strawberries (two cups, should be about 10 ounces)
- One small banana
- A bunch of fresh spinach (two cups or more)
- One pomegranate
- Flaxseeds (one tablespoon)
- Ice cubes

Directions

1. Remove the seeds in the pomegranate and place them in a blender. Add the remaining ingredients.

2. Add ice to fill it up, then set the blender to high speed and puree until it's smooth.
3. Pour into two glasses and enjoy. Best served with a straw.

GINGER TEA

Ingredients

- 2 sprigs dill weed
- 2 tbsp fresh lime juice
- 4 cups spring water
- A pinch of cayenne
- One thumb of fresh ginger root (make sure it's organic; you can also substitute with powder garlic)
- Raw agave to taste (optional)

Instructions

1. Start by boiling the water.
2. Next, peel and chop the ginger root. Then add it to the pot of boiling water followed by the weed.
3. Cook for about 5 minutes, then strain the tea into a glass jar or bowl. Add the lime juice and stir. Finally, add the cayenne and agave. Stir again.
4. Serve either hot or cold.

QUINOA PORRIDGE

Ingredients

- ½ cup coconut milk or cream
- 1 cup dry quinoa
- ½ tsp cayenne
- ½ lime, with skin grated
- 2 cups water (ideally, spring water)
- Half a handful of assorted nuts and seeds
- Ground cloves to taste

Instructions

1. First make the quinoa by following the instructions on the package.
2. Next, drain the quinoa, then pour it into a saucepan. Add the cloves and cayenne. Combine everything.
3. Add the milk and grated lime. Optionally, add grated apple.
4. Top with seeds and nuts. Serve.

PECAN, COCONUT & OATMEAL

Ingredients

- Half a cup of coconut or almond milk
- One tablespoon of coconut flakes
- ¼ teaspoon of pure vanilla extract
- ¼ teaspoon of ground cinnamon

- Two tablespoons of almond flour
- Two tablespoons of hemp hearts
- Two teaspoons of chia seeds
- One tablespoon of flax meal
- One tablespoon of pecans, toasted and chopped

Instructions

1. Combine the chia seeds, flax meal, almond flour, cinnamon, vanilla, hemp hearts, and milk in a small pot. Cook over low heat, stirring occasionally until the mixture becomes thick. This should take about 5 minutes.

2. Spoon everything into a bowl or dish and top with coconut flakes and pecans. Serve immediately.

AVOCADO & MUNG BEAN SPROUTS SALAD

Ingredients

- Sea salt to taste
- 1 to 2 avocados, diced
- One lime, juiced
- One cup of mung bean sprouts
- Fresh basil
- 1 to 2 tomatoes, cubed
- ¼ cup of olive oil

Instructions

1. Combine all the ingredients in a small bowl. Mix well and serve.

TROPICAL GAZPACHO

Ingredients
- 1½ cups of organic tomato juice

- Salt and pepper
- Tabasco (optional, optional)
- Half a cup of cucumber (peeled, seeded, and chopped)
- Orange ball pepper (half cup, chopped)
- Half small red onion (peeled and chopped)
- Chopped mango (one cup)
- Chopped papaya (one cup)
- Chopped pineapple (half cup)
- Minced cilantro ($1/8$ cup, fresh)

Directions
1. Put all the ingredients in a blender. Puree them, then transfer to a large bowl and season to taste.
2. Put it in a refrigerator to get cold. Serve and enjoy!

MUESLI WITH NUTS & DRIED FRUIT

Ingredients

- Muesli cereal (half cup)

- Raisins (one tablespoon)
- Half cup of almond milk (you can substitute with low-fat rice or brown rice)
- One teaspoon of almonds (sliced or slivered)
- Walnuts (one teaspoon, chopped)
- Dried berries (one tablespoon, mixed)

Directions

1. Pour the milk and cereal into a bowl to mix them. Add more milk if it's too thick.
2. Use the raisins, walnuts, almonds, and berries as toppings. Serve ASAP.

ALMOND BUTTER AND WHOLE GRAIN BREAD

Ingredients

- Almond butter (one tablespoon)
- Whole Grain Bread (one slice)
- Half medium pear (peeled, cored, sliced)

- Chopped walnuts (one teaspoon)

Directions

1. Spread the butter over the bread. Then place the sliced pears on top.
2. Sprinkle with walnuts. Enjoy!

GREEN AVOCADO SMOOTHIE

Ingredients

- Half a cup of spring water
- Two tablespoons of sea moss gel
- One fresh avocado
- One organic burro banana
- Natural sweetener (optional, example is stevia)

Instructions

1. Start by peeling the banana and avocado.

2. Add to a blender together with the sea moss gel, sweetener, and water. Blend until smooth.

DR SEBI BREAKFAST HERBAL SMOOTHIE

Ingredient

- 1 tbsp agave syrup (or stevia)
- 1 blow banana, peeled
- 1 tbsp walnuts
- 2 cups Dr Sebi Herbal Tea

Instructions

1. Add the ingredients to a blender and pulse for a minute until smooth.
2. Transfer the drink into one or two glasses and enjoy!

EASY CLEANSING TEA

Ingredients

- One teaspoon of prodigiosa powder
- One cup of spring water
- One teaspoon of burdock root powder

Instructions

1. Put the ingredients in a tea kettle and boil for ten minutes.
2. Remove from heat, cover and leave it for another ten minutes. Drain and serve.

SPICY KALE

Ingredient

- ¼ cup red pepper, diced

- ¼ tsp sea salt
- 1 tsp red pepper, crushed
- ¼ cup diced onion
- 1 cup kale leaves, chopped
- 2 tbsp grapeseed oil

Instructions

1. Start by heating the grapeseed oil in a pan. Once the oil gets hot, add the diced onion and pepper and saute for about two to three minutes. Next, season with salt.
2. Lower the heat. Then pour in the kale leaves. Cover the pan and simmer for about 5 minutes.
3. Remove the cover and add in the crushed pepper. Stir well, then cover again. Let it cool for about 4 minutes. Serve!

ALKALINE MILLET

Ingredients

- 2 ½ cups water
- 1 cup millet
- ½ tsp sea salt

Instructions

1. First thing is to saute the millet until golden brown. Then add water and salt.
2. Bring the mixture to a boil then simmer for about 30 minutes or until the water is absorbed.
3. Remove from heat and allow to cool with the lid still on. Serve!

TASTY PANINI

Ingredients

- One ripe banana, chopped
- Two slices whole grain bread
- ¼ cup natural peanut butter
- ¼ cup hot water
- ¼ cup raisin
- 1 tsp cinnamon
- 2 tsp cacao powder

Instructions

1. In a bowl, combine the hot water, cinnamon, and cacao powder. Mix well.
2. Next, spread the butter on the bread slices.
3. Place the chopped bananas on the toast.
4. Now, combine the raisin and mixture from step 1 in a blender and spread it on the sandwich.

ROASTED TOMATO AND BELL PEPPER SOUP

Ingredients

- Five tomatoes (choose large ones)
- Three large red bell pepper (quartered, seeded)
- 4-6 garlic cloves (peeled)
- Olive oil (two teaspoons)
- Thyme (one teaspoon, fresh & minced)
- Fresh minced basil (two tablespoons)
- Vegetable stock (two cups, make sure it's low in fat and sodium)
- Salt & pepper to taste

Directions

1. Start by preheating the oven. Set it to 450 degrees Fahrenheit.
2. Get an oiled baking sheet. Place the peppers, garlic, and tomatoes on the sheet.
3. Next, drizzle olive oil over the vegetables and roast for half an hour or until they become brownish.
4. Take the vegetables out from the oven and let it cool. Then puree them in a blender.

5. Next transfer the pureed vegetables to a saucepan, then add your thyme and stock and bring to soup consistency.
6. Now, pour in the basil and boil. Use medium heat.
7. The soup is best served cold!

SOUTHERN ONION SOUP

Ingredients

- Three tablespoons of olive oil
- Two cups sweet onions, thinly sliced (such as Vidalia)
- One dash of nutmeg
- One 10 ½ oz package of soft silken tofu
- Four cups of salted vegetable stock (if stock is not salted, you can add half a teaspoon of salt)

Instructions

1. Start by sautéing the onions and olive oil in a skillet until transparent over medium heat.
2. Pour the vegetable stock into a saucepan and add in the sautéd onions. Cover the saucepan and simmer for 25 to 30 minutes or until the onions become very soft.
3. Remove the saucepan from heat and pour the soup into a blender. Optionally, break a block of soft tofu into smaller pieces and add to the soup in the blender.
4. Now, blend for two to three minutes or until smooth.
5. Finally, transfer the soup in the blender into dishes and garnish with a dash of nutmeg. Serve hot or chilled.

EASY TEFF PORRIDGE

Ingredients

- ½ cup teff grain

- 2 cups of water (ideally, spring water)
- A pinch of salt
- Blueberries and agave nectar to taste

Ingredients

1. Pour the water into a saucepan and bring to a boil. Then add the salt and teff grain. Stir thoroughly.
2. Reduce the heat to low heat and simmer for 15 minutes with the lid on.
3. Serve with blueberries and agave as toppings.

EASY FRUIT SALAD

Ingredients

- One pint of fresh strawberries, sliced without stems
- One pint of fresh blueberries
- Two cups of grapes
- One ripe pear, cored and diced

- Two tablespoons of date syrup, optional
- ¼ tsp ground cinnamon

Instructions

1. Combine all the ingredients in a bowl. Stir to mix well.
2. Keep in the refrigerator and serve chill.

HERBERT HUMMUS

Ingredients

- ¼ cup of chives, chopped
- Half a cup of fresh tarragon leaves, blanched with light packing
- Two garlic cloves
- One cup of fresh basil leaves, blanched with light packing

- Four cups of garbanzo beans, cooked
- Freshly squeezed juice from one lemon
- One cup of vegetable broth
- Half a cup of fresh flat parsley leaves
- Two tablespoons of sesame seeds, toasted

Instructions

1. Start by dabbing the basil leaves and tarragon until dry. Then cut into smaller sizes and add to a blender.
2. Next, also add the lemon juice, beans, sesame seeds, garlic, lemon juice, and vegetable broth to the blender. Blend until smooth and creamy.

Add chives and stir. Enjoy.

ELECTRIC SALAD

Ingredients

- Olive oil
- 1 cup cherry tomatoes
- 1 cup kale, chopped
- 2 red onions
- 3 Jalapenos
- A handful of romaine lettuce
- Juice from 1 lime
- 1 orange pepper
- 1 yellow pepper

Directions

1. Wash and rinse the ingredients. After drying, cut into smaller bite-sized pieces.
2. Put everything in a bowl, then drizzle with the olive oil and lemon juice. Enjoy!

EASY VEGETABLE BROTH

Ingredients

- Eight cups of water
- Three ribs of celery, chopped
- Five cloves of garlic, minced
- Three carrots, chopped
- Two bay leaves
- Two to three cups of vegetable scraps, frozen
- Two large onions, chopped
- A few sprigs of thyme
- A few sprigs of parsley
- One tablespoon of olive oil
- Salt and pepper to taste

Instructions

1. Start by heating the olive oil in a large stockpot or Dutch oven over medium heat.
2. Once the oil is hot, add in the onions, carrots, and celery and cook until softened. This should take about 5 minutes. Make sure to stir frequently.
3. Next, add the water and the remaining ingredients - bay leaves, thyme, parsley, and frozen vegetable

scraps. Reduce the stove to low heat and simmer for about 45 minutes with the pot partially covered.

4. Now, pour the broth through a fine mesh strainer into another large pot or bowl. You can discard the solids.

5. Allow the broth to cool, then pour it into freezer bags or airtight containers and keep in the freezer until you're ready to use it.

GRANOLA

Ingredients

- Honey (¼ cup)
- Grapeseed oil (¼ cup)
- Cinnamon (two teaspoons)
- Almond extract (one teaspoon)
- Orange extract (one teaspoon)
- Rolled oats (three and half cups)
- Slivered almonds (¼ cup)
- Walnuts (¼ cup, chopped)

Directions

1. Preheat the oven. The temperature should be 350 degrees Fahrenheit.
2. Pour the honey into a bowl, then add all the extracts, oil, and spices.
3. Add the nuts and oats and stir well.
4. Now, spread the mixture over a greased cookie sheet. Bake for ten minutes, then stir and continue

to bake for another 10 minutes or until the mixture turns golden brown.

5. Let it cool, then you can break it apart. Put into a container for storage. The container should be airtight. Enjoy!
6. This can be topped with fruits and enjoyed with your favorite plant-based milk drink such as low-fat soy milk or almond oil.
7. To make things more interesting, you can add a teaspoon of freshly grounded flaxseeds to each serving.

BERRY BREAKFAST SHAKE

Ingredients

- Half a teaspoon of lemon juice, freshly squeezed
- ¼ cup of mixed berries, frozen
- Half a cup of almond milk or coconut milk

- Half a cup of heavy cream
- One tablespoon of MCT oil (optional)
- One tablespoon of almond butter

Instructions

1. Add all the ingredients to a blender and blend until you get a smooth consistency. Serve immediately.

CHOCOLATE AND PEANUT BUTTER SHAKE

Ingredients

- ½ cup plant-based yogurt
- ¾ cup frozen banana, sliced
- One tablespoon natural peanut butter
- One cup of vanilla soy milk, unsweetened
- One tablespoon of cocoa powder

Directions

1. Combine everything in a blender and blend until smooth. Enjoy!

Conclusion

I will draw the curtains here.

Managing IBD through your diet shouldn't be overwhelming. All it requires is a personalized approach with an emphasis on maintaining a balanced diet and avoiding trigger foods that can exacerbate your symptoms.

Overall, a nutrient-dense diet focused on whole grains, fruits, vegetables, and plant proteins will not only provide relief but also aid recovery and support your gut health. This is what a plant diet aims to achieve.

However, it's worth mentioning that following the right diet is not enough. For a long-lasting solution, you need a more holistic approach, which means paying attention to your lifestyle and addressing areas that impact your overall health.

www.ingramcontent.com/pod-product-compliance
Lightning Source LLC
Chambersburg PA
CBHW070416230526
45471CB00006B/2838